Vegetarian Essential Recipes

A Handful of Quick, Delicious Recipes for Your

Vegetarian Meals

Lea Tanner

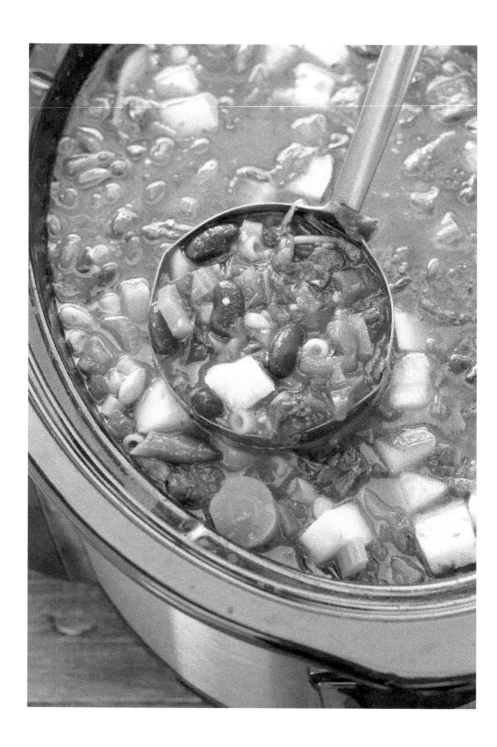

implied. Readers acknowledge that the author is not engaging in the rendering of legal, financial, medical or professional advice. The content within this book has been derived from various sources. Please consult a licensed professional before attempting any techniques outlined in this book.

By reading this document, the reader agrees that under no circumstances is the author responsible for any losses, direct or indirect, which are incurred as a result of the use of information contained within this document, including, but not limited to, — errors, omissions, or inaccuracies.

Table of Contents

Nettle Soup

Yum! This is really wonderful and super easy to make soup

Ingredients:

1½ cups of nettle leaves, blanched

2 large potatoes, peeled and cubed

1 onion, chopped finely

2 cloves of garlic, chopped

Salt, to taste

5 cups of water

1 cup of milk

1½ tablespoons of flour

3 tablespoons of butter

Black pepper, to taste

A pinch of nutmeg powder

Directions:

In a pan, add nettle, potatoes, onion, garlic, 1 teaspoon of salt and water. Bring to a boil on medium-high heat. Reduce heat to medium-low. Simmer for 25 to 30 minutes or till potatoes become tender. Let it cool slightly.

Add soup in a food processor and blend till smooth. Transfer the soup to the pan again.

Pour milk and mix well. In a bowl, add flour and butter and whisk till smooth. Add 1 cup of soup and mix well. Add the flour mixture in soup pan. Cook, stirring often for 5 minutes on medium-low heat.

Remove from stove and stir in desired salt, pepper and nutmeg.

Serving suggestions:

It will be a major hit if this soup is served with sour cream and roasted and chopped walnuts.

Celery Soup

A simple, delicious and fabulous soup that even those people will love who do not like celery.

Ingredients:

2 tablespoons of butter

1 large onion, chopped

4 cups of celery, chopped

2 (14 ½-ounce) cans of low-sodium vegetable broth

1 large russet potato, peeled and cubed

1 pound of celery roots, peeled and cut into 1-inch pieces

2 cloves of garlic, chopped

½ teaspoon of celery salt

1 cup of cream, whipped

Salt and black pepper, to taste

Directions:

In a pan, melt butter on medium heat. Add onion and celery and cook, stirring often for about 20 minutes.

Add broth, potatoes, celery roots, garlic and salt. Bring to a boil. Reduce heat to medium-low. Cover and simmer for 30 minutes or till vegetables become very tender. Remove from stove. Let it cool slightly.

Add soup in a food processor and blend till smooth. Transfer soup to pan again. Stir in cream. Bring to a boil, stirring occasionally.

Season with salt and pepper.

Serving Suggestions:

This soup is great with corn bread.

Black Bean Soup

A yummy soup with zesty flavor!! Even your picky kids will love this soup.

Ingredients:

1 tablespoon of vegetable oil

1 medium onion, chopped

1 teaspoon of cumin powder

1 teaspoon of chili powder

¼ teaspoon of salsa, prepared

¼ teaspoon of salt

3 cups of water

2 (15-ounce) cans of black beans, rinsed and drained

1 tablespoon of fresh lime juice

Directions:

In a pan, heat oil on medium heat. Sauté onion for 2 minutes. Stir in cumin and chili powder and cook for 1 minute further. Add salsa, salt, water and beans. Reduce heat to medium-low. Simmer for 10 minutes.

Remove from stove. Add lime juice. Add soup in food processor and puree till smooth.

Transfer soup to pan again. Heat the soup gently.

Garnish cilantro while serving.

Serving Suggestions:

Enjoy this yummy soup with tortilla chips.

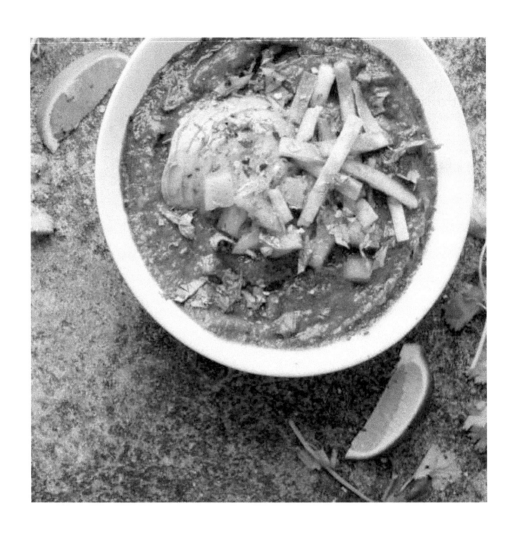

Vegetarian Barley Soup

Easy to prepare and tasty!! Barley, vegetables and broth make this soup healthy and hearty.

Ingredients:

2 tablespoons of canola oil

1 medium onion, chopped

2 celery stalks, diced into ¼-inch size

2 carrots, diced into ¼-inch size

1 clove of garlic

1 cup of pearl barley

4 cups of vegetable broth

2 plum tomatoes, chopped

4 sprigs of fresh thyme, chopped

2 bay leaves

Salt and black pepper, to taste

Directions:

In a pan, heat oil on medium-high heat. Sauté onion till translucent.

Add celery, carrots and garlic. Cook till vegetables become soft. Add barley, broth, tomatoes, thyme and bay leaves.

Reduce heat to medium-low. Simmer for about 30 minutes or till barley becomes soft.

Season with salt and black pepper.

Serving Suggestions:

Serve this tasty soup with crusty bread.

Pear Salad

It's beautiful, awesome and composed pear salad as side dish.

Ingredients:

For Salad:

1 large pear, sliced thinly

1 bunch of lettuce, torn

½ cup of dried cranberries

¼ cup of Swiss cheese, grated

1 cup of pecans, toasted

For Vinaigrette:

¼ cup of olive oil

¼ cup of lemon juice

1 teaspoon of prepared mustard

½ cup of sugar

½ teaspoon of salt

2 teaspoons of red onion, chopped finely

2 teaspoons of poppy seeds

Directions:

In a large bowl, add pear, lettuce, cranberries, cheese and pecans and mix well. In another bowl, add all vinaigrette ingredients and whisk till well combined. Pour over salad and toss to coat well.

Serving suggestions:

Enhance the flavor of this awesome salad by drizzling with some maple syrup.

Quinoa & Black Bean Salad

This flavorful salad has also the potential to be a main course.

Ingredients:

For Salad:

1 cup of red quinoa

2 cups of water

1 (15-ounce) can of corn kernels, drained

1 (15-ounce) can of black beans, rinsed and drained

¼ cup of fresh cilantro, chopped

1 scallion, chopped

1 jalapeño pepper, diced

½ red pepper diced

For Dressing:

1 tablespoon of extra-virgin olive oil

1 tablespoon of lime juice

½ teaspoon of chipotle powder

Salt and black pepper, to taste

1 teaspoon of cumin powder

Directions:

In a pan, add quinoa and water. Bring to a boil on medium-high heat. Reduce heat to medium-low. Simmer for 20 minutes or till all liquid is absorbed.

In a large bowl, fluff quinoa with fork. In the same bowl, add corn, black beans, cilantro, scallion, jalapeño and red pepper and mix well.

In another bowl, add all dressing ingredients and whisk till well mixed.

Pour dressing on salad and toss till well coated.

Serving Suggestions:

If you like spicier flavor then you can add hot sauce in dressing.

Green Bean Salad

This yummy and fresh salad has a creamy texture of cheese and crunch of green beans.

Ingredients:

½ cup of shallots, chopped finely

1½ pounds of fresh green beans, trimmed and cut into 2-inch pieces

¾ cup of fresh basil leaves, chopped

4 tablespoons of extra-virgin olive oil

2 tablespoons of balsamic vinegar

Salt and black pepper, to taste

¾ cup of Parmesan cheese, grated fresh

Directions:

Add shallots in a water filled bowl and keep aside. Add water in a large pan and bring to a boil. Add beans and blanch for almost 2 minutes.

In the mean time fill a bowl with ice water. Transfer beans from boiled water to ice water. Drain shallots and beans well. In a large bowl, add shallots, beans and basil and mix.

Pour oil and vinegar and toss well.

Now add salt, black pepper and cheese. Toss till well coated.

Chill salad before serving.

Serving Suggestions:

You can serve this fresh salad with toasted walnuts or pecans.

Vegetarian Taco Salad

This salad is so bright and colorful and also rich in flavors.

Ingredients:

2 tablespoons of extra-virgin olive oil

1½ cups of frozen corn kernels, thawed

1 large onion, chopped

1 large tomato, chopped plus 3 large tomatoes, chopped coarsely

¼ teaspoon of salt

1½ teaspoons of dried oregano, divided

1 (15-ounce) can of black beans, rinsed

1 tablespoon of chili powder

1/3 cup of salsa, prepared

½ cup of fresh cilantro, chopped

2 cups of lettuce, chopped

1½ cups of long-grain brown rice, cooked

1 cup of pepper jack cheese, grated

Lime wedges, as requires

2½ cups of tortilla chips, crumbled coarsely

Directions:

In a large pan, heat oil on medium heat. Add corn and onion. Cook, stirring for 5 minutes.

Add beans, rice, 1 tomato, salt, 1 teaspoon of oregano and chili powder. Cook, stirring often for 5 minutes or till tomato cooks completely. Keep aside for cooling.

In a bowl, add 3 tomatoes, remaining oregano, salsa and cilantro and mix well.

In another bowl, add bean mixture, salsa mixture and lettuce.

Toss till coated well. Sprinkle cheese, lime wedges and tortilla chips.

Serving Suggestions:

You can toast the tortilla chips for more crispy touch.

Cucumber, Avocado & Tomato Salad

The fresh flavors of this salad are perfect for summer.

Ingredients:

2 cucumbers, sliced into bite size pieces

4 tomatoes, sliced into bite size pieces

2 avocadoes, sliced into bite size pieces

½ cup of cilantro. Chopped finely

1 tablespoon of olive oil

2 tablespoons of fresh lime juice

Salt and black pepper, to taste

Directions:

In a bowl, mix cucumber, tomatoes, avocado and cilantro.

Pour oil and lemon juice on salad.

Season with salt and black pepper. Toss to coat well.

Serving Suggestions:

This fresh salad is great as snack if served with pita chips.

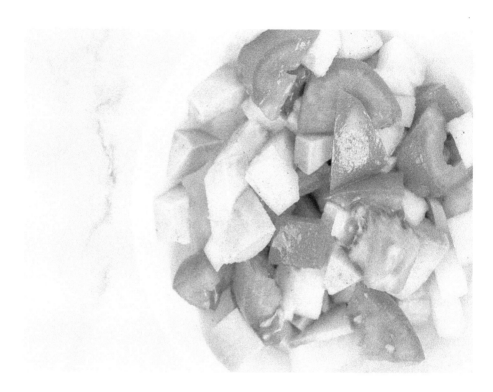

Tomato & Goat Cheese Bruschetta

Delicious and elegant!! This is a very simple way to make a nice appetizer.

Ingredients:

1 loaf of Italian bread, sliced diagonally into ½-inch thick size

2 cloves of garlic cut in half

3 tablespoons of olive oil, divided

1 package of soft goat cheese, cut into 1-inch slices

¼ teaspoon of fresh black pepper powder

1 teaspoon of fresh oregano leaves, chopped finely

2 medium tomatoes, seeded and diced

2 teaspoons of fresh parsley leaves, chopped finely and divided

Salt, to taste

Directions:

Prepare grill on medium heat. Grill bread slices for 3 to 4 minutes from both sides. Rub one side of slice with garlic. Brush with olive oil.

In a bowl, add goat cheese, black pepper and oregano. Mix till well blended.

In another bowl, add tomatoes, 1 teaspoon of parsley, remaining oil and salt and toss to coat.

Place goat cheese mixture on toasted slices. Place tomato mixture on top. Sprinkle remaining parsley.

Serving Suggestions:

Enjoy your cheesy brochette with fresh salad.

Hummus Bruschetta

This tasty bruschetta looks great to entertain guests in party.

Ingredients:

1 (14-ounce) can of chickpeas, drained

¼ teaspoon of garlic, chopped

2 teaspoons of olive oil

3 tablespoons of lemon juice

¼ teaspoon of cumin powder

12 slices of ciabatta slices

4 tablespoons of butter, softened

¼ cup of Parmesan cheese, grated fresh

1 teaspoon of paprika

½ cup of feta cheese, crumbled

2 tablespoons of kalamata olives, pitted and sliced

24 slices of plum tomatoes

Fresh oregano, chopped for garnishing

Directions:

Preheat oven to 325 degrees F.

In a food processor, add chickpeas, garlic, oil, lemon juice and cumin powder. Pulse for 1 minute or till well mixed. Refrigerate hummus overnight for best flavor. Bring to room temperature before using.

Spread butter on each slice evenly. Sprinkle Parmesan cheese on each slice. Place slices in oven under broiler for about 3 minutes. Remove from oven.

In a bowl, mix feta cheese, olives and tomatoes. Spread hummus on each slice evenly. Sprinkle paprika. Place tomatoes mixture on top. Garnish with chopped oregano.

Serving Suggestions:

You can serve these tasty bruschetta with avocado dip.

Mushroom Bruschetta

Great recipe! It is super easy and tasty starter.

Ingredients:

6 slices of Italian bread, sliced

3 tablespoons of olive oil plus extra

4 cloves of garlic, chopped finely

1 pound of Portobello mushrooms, chopped

Salt and black pepper, to taste

2 tablespoons of fresh thyme leaves, chopped

2 tablespoons of fresh parsley leaves, chopped

Directions:

Preheat grill. Toast the slices on grill for 3 to 4 minutes from each side.

In a pan, heat oil on medium-high. Sauté garlic till fragrant. Add mushrooms, salt and pepper. Pour a little olive oil in pan. Reduce heat to medium. Cook, stirring occasionally for about 10 to 12 minutes.

Stir in thyme and parsley and cook for 5 more minutes.

mushroom mixture on bread slices.

Serving Suggestions:

Serve with tomato relish for more taste.

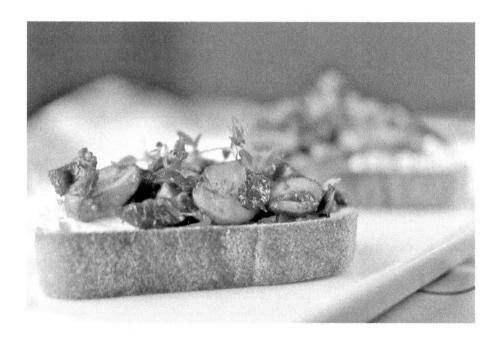

Apple & Pear Bruschetta

This combination sounds fantastic for a light meal.

Ingredients:

8 slices of crusty bread

3 ounces of goat cheese, cut into 1-inch slices

1 Fuji apple, peeled and sliced thinly

1 pear, sliced thinly

2 to 3 tablespoons of honey

3 tablespoons of almonds, toasted and sliced

Directions:

Preheat the grill. Lightly toast the slices for 3 to 4 minutes each side.

In a bowl, mix apple and pear. Spread cheese on bread slices. Place fruit mixture on cheese. Drizzle honey over fruit. Top with toasted almonds.

Serving Suggestions:

You can replace the cheese of your choice as blue cheese or brie cheese.

Garlic Veggie Bruschetta

Decent and colorful veggie bruschetta....

Ingredients:

1 tablespoon of olive oil

2 cloves of garlic, chopped finely

1 zucchini, cubed

1 eggplant, cubed

1 tomato, skinned, seeded and chopped

Salt and black pepper, to taste

1 tablespoon of fresh basil, chopped

1 tablespoon of fresh oregano, chopped

1 loaf of baguette, cut into 1-inch thick slices

6 teaspoons of butter, softened

4 teaspoons of garlic powder

Directions:

Preheat oven to 325 degrees F.

In a skillet, heat oil on medium heat. Sauté garlic for about 2 minutes. Add zucchini and eggplant. Cook for 5 to 7 minutes.

Add tomatoes and stir till tomato becomes pulpy. Stir in salt, black pepper, basil and oregano.

Cook for 2 more minutes. Spread butter on each slice evenly. Sprinkle garlic powder. Place the slices on oven rack and bake for 3 to 4 minutes.

Transfer slices to a plate. Place vegetable mixture on slices evenly.

Serving Suggestions:

If you are a cheese lover then top vegetables with grated mozzarella cheese.

Applesauce Bread

This quick, moist and fragrant nutty bread is great in lunch boxes for your little ones.

Ingredients:

2½ cups of flour, sifted

1 tablespoon of baking powder

2 tablespoons of cinnamon powder

¼ teaspoon of salt

1 large egg

2/3 cup of fat-free milk

1 cup of light brown sugar

2 tablespoons of vegetable oil

1 cup of applesauce

½ cup of raisins

1 cup of walnuts, chopped and divided

Directions:

Preheat oven to 350 degrees F. Grease a loaf pan.

In a bowl, add flour, salt, baking powder and cinnamon. In another bowl, beat egg. Add milk, sugar, oil and applesauce. Stir till well mixed. Mix flour mixture and egg mixture till combined. Stir in raisins and ½ cup of walnuts.

Place batter in prepared loaf pan. Sprinkle remaining walnuts on top. Bake for 55 to 60 minutes or till a toothpick inserted in center comes out clean.

Let it cool in pan for 10 minutes. Remove from pan and let it cool completely.

Serving Suggestions:

Spread peanut butter on bread slices and enjoy.

Zucchini Bread

Make this zucchini bread and surely you will have a flavorful, tasty and sweet snack for breakfast or teatime.

Ingredients:

1½ cups of all-purpose flour, sifted

¼ teaspoon of baking soda

1 teaspoons of baking powder

½ teaspoon of salt

Nutmeg powder, to taste

1 teaspoon of cinnamon powder

1 large egg

½ cup of vegetable oil

¼ cup of packed brown sugar

½ cup of white sugar

1 teaspoon of vanilla extract

½ pound of zucchini trimmed, grated and squeezed completely

½ cup of walnuts, chopped

½ cup of raisins

Directions:

Preheat the oven to 350 degrees F. Grease a loaf pan.

In a bowl, add flour, baking soda, baking powder, salt, nutmeg and cinnamon and mix well. In another bowl, add egg, oil, brown sugar, white sugar, vanilla extract and beat till combined.

Add zucchini, walnut and raisins in flour mixture and toss well. Mix flour mixture and egg mixture.

Place batter in loaf pan. Bake for 40 to 45 minutes or till a toothpick inserted in center comes out clean.

Let it cool in pan for 10 minutes. Remove from pan and let it cool completely.

Serving Suggestions:

While serving, spread some butter on slices and sprinkle a little powdered sugar and chocolate chips and have more taste.

Cinnamon Rolls

These delicious rolls rock! A great snack for friends at teatime....

Ingredients:

For Rolls:

2½ cups of all-purpose flour, plus extra for dusting

½ teaspoon of baking soda

1¼ teaspoon of baking powder

6 tablespoons of granulated sugar, divided

Salt, to taste

¾ cup of light brown sugar

Nutmeg powder, to taste

2½ teaspoons of cinnamon powder

8 tablespoons of butter, melted

1¼ cup of buttermilk

For Glaze:

3 tablespoons of butter, softened

3 ounces of cream cheese, softened

1 cup of powdered sugar

¼ teaspoon of vanilla extract

¼ cup of milk

Directions:

Preheat oven to 425 degrees F. Grease a baking pan.

In a bowl, add flour, baking soda, baking powder, 2 tablespoons of granulated sugar and ½ teaspoon of salt and mix well.

In second bowl, remaining granulated sugar, nutmeg, cinnamon, a pinch of salt and 1 tablespoon of butter and whisk till well combined. Add 2 tablespoons of butter in buttermilk and mix well.

Stir in buttermilk mixture in flour mixture till a dough forms. Knead the dough till smooth. Dust flour on plain surface. With your hands, pat the dough into a rectangle shape.

Spread melted butter on dough evenly. Sprinkle cinnamon mixture and press into the dough.

Roll the dough and pinch the ends to seal. Cut the rolled dough in equal parts.

Place the rolls in prepared baking pan. Brush the rolls with remaining butter.

Bake for 23 to 25 minutes or till the edges become golden brown.

While rolls are in oven for baking, prepare glaze. In a bowl, mix butter and cream cheese and beat till fluffy. Mix remaining ingredients till well combined.

Pour glaze on warm rolls and serve.

Serving Suggestions:

Enjoy these delicious rolls with coffee or tea.

Blueberry & Raspberry Muffins

Add these tasty and luxurious but healthy muffins to your gourmet morning menu.

Ingredients:

1 cup of all-propose flour, sifted

½ teaspoon of baking soda

1 teaspoon of baking powder

½ teaspoon of salt

1 cup of sour cream

2 eggs

5 tablespoons of butter

1 cup of light brown sugar

1 cup of rolled oats

½ cup of raspberries

½ cup of blueberries

1 tablespoon of powdered sugar

Directions:

Preheat oven to 375 degrees F. Line one (12-cups) muffin tray with wax paper.

In a bowl, mix flour, baking soda, baking powder and salt. Keep aside.

In a second bowl, add sour cream and egg and whisk till well mixed.

In a pan, melt butter and brown sugar on medium heat. Let it cool slightly. Mix in egg mixture. Stir in oats. Mix flour mixture and egg mixture till well combined. Gently fold in berries.

Dollop the batter into muffin cups. Sprinkle powdered sugar on all muffin cups. Bake for 20 to 25 minutes or till tops become firm and edges are light brown.

Let it cool for 5 minutes. Then transfer muffins into paper cups.

Sprinkle powdered sugar on all muffins.

Serving Suggestions:

These yummy muffins are perfect with a cup of tea.

Carrot Cake Muffins

These carrot-filled muffins with creamy top are ideal for breakfast or lunch box treat.

Ingredients:

For Muffins:

2¼ cups of all-purpose flour

¼ teaspoon of baking soda

1½ teaspoon of baking powder

¼ cup of light brown sugar

½ cup of granulated sugar

¾ teaspoon of salt

¾ teaspoon of ginger powder

1½ teaspoons of cinnamon powder

2 large eggs

1/3 cup of vegetable oil

¾ cup of water

1 cup of carrots, grated

For frosting:

1 (8-ounce) package of cream cheese

¼ teaspoon of vanilla extract

¼ cup of granulated sugar

Directions:

Preheat oven to 400 degrees F. Grease one (12-cups) muffin tray.

In a bowl, mix flour, brown sugar, ginger, baking soda, baking powder, granulated sugar, salt and cinnamon.

In another bowl, add eggs, oil and water and whisk well. Add egg mixture in flour mixture and mix well. Stir in carrots and mix well.

For frosting, microwave cream cheese for 40 seconds. Stir in vanilla extract and sugar.

Place muffin batter in muffin cups. Pour a tablespoon of cream cheese mixture on top. Bake for about 20 minutes or till a toothpick inserted in center of muffins, comes out clean.

Remove muffin tray from oven. Let it cool for 5 minutes.

Transfer muffins to paper cups and serve.

Serving Suggestions:

If you like nuts then garnish muffins with toasted nuts of your choice.

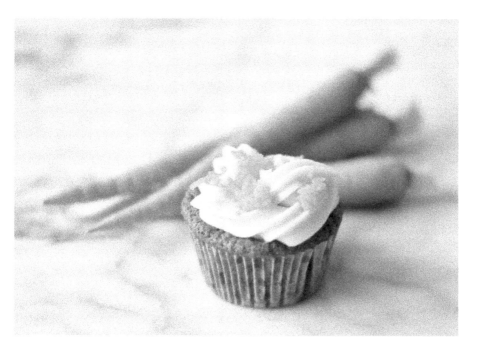

Avocado & Sun-Dried Tomato Sandwich

One of best summer lunches!

Ingredients:

1 ripe avocado, halved and pitted

2 tablespoons of light sour cream

1 clove of garlic, minced

1 tablespoon of lemon juice

Salt and pepper, to taste

5 to 6 oil packed sun-dried tomatoes, sliced thinly

1½ tablespoons of oil from sun-dried tomatoes

4 lettuce leaves, washed and pat dried

4 slices of bread

Directions:

With a spoon, scoop out avocado pulp. Mash with a fork.

In a bowl, mix avocado, sour cream, garlic, lemon juice, salt and pepper.

Brush the slices with oil. Place lettuce leaves on 2 slices of bread. Spread avocado mixture on lettuce leaves. Place tomato slices on avocado mixture. Close each sandwich with other slices of bread.

Serving Suggestions:

These sandwiches go nice with soup of your choice.

Hummus with Grated Carrots & Radish Sandwich

A terrific, lovely and healthy sandwich with vegetables and hummus!

Ingredients:

For Hummus:

1 (14-ounce) can of chickpeas, drained

½ teaspoon of garlic, chopped

2 tablespoons of olive oil

3 tablespoons of lemon juice

1 teaspoon of cumin powder

1/3 cup of sesame seed paste

3 tablespoons of water

3 tablespoons of fresh parsley, minced

For Sandwich:

1 large carrot, grated

½ cup of radish, grated

½ cup of cucumber, seeded and sliced

½ cup of alfalfa sprouts plus extra for garnishing

1 small sweet onion, sliced thinly

1½ tablespoons of sesame seeds, toasted

6 slices of wheat bread

Directions:

In a food processor, add all hummus ingredients and pulse till smooth. Refrigerate hummus overnight for better taste. Bring to room temperature before use.

In a bowl combine all vegetables and sesame seeds.

Spread hummus on bread slices. Place vegetable mixture on hummus. Close each sandwich with another slice of bread, hummus side down.

Cut in half and serve.

Serving Suggestions:

This can also be served as a snack if paired with tortilla chips.

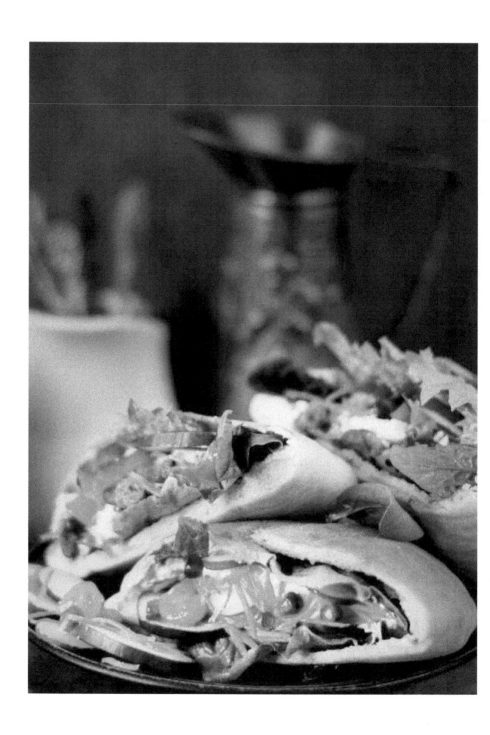

Peanut Butter & Apple Slices Sandwich

These sandwiches are a simple but impressive combination of flavors.

Ingredients:

4 slices of whole-grain bread

4 tablespoons of peanut butter

2 Granny Smith apples, peeled, cored and sliced thinly

Directions:

Spread a thick layer of peanut butter on bread slices. Place apple slices on peanut butter. Close sandwich with other slice, peanut butter side down.

Cut in half and serve.

Serving Suggestions:

These delicious sandwiches are great with a glass of cold milk.

Cucumber, Tomato & Goat Cheese Sandwich

Refreshing and healthy sandwiches which are easy to handle......

Ingredients:

½ cucumber, sliced thinly

2 medium tomatoes, sliced thinly

2 tablespoons of lettuce leaves, chopped

¼ cup of walnuts, toasted and chopped

Salt and pepper, to taste

4 slices of whole-grain bread

½ (4-ounce) log of goat cheese, at room temperature

Directions:

In a bowl, add cucumber, tomato, lettuce leaves, walnuts, salt and pepper and toss well.

Spread goat cheese on all slices.

Place veggie mixture on peanut butter.

Top with other slices, keeping cheese side down.

Lastly to serve, cut in half and serve.

Serving Suggestions:

Enjoy your sandwiches with pasta salad.

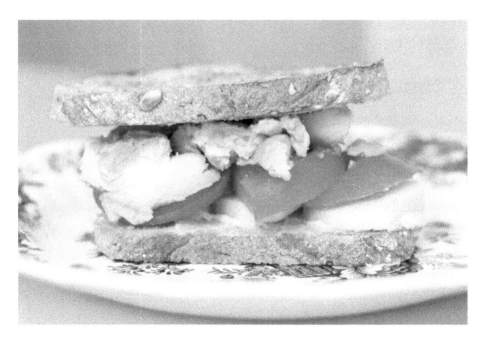

Grilled Portobello, Mozzarella & Olive Oil Sandwich

Surely these sandwiches will be a huge hit for your family.

Ingredients:

4 tablespoons of olive oil plus extra for greasing

1 red bell pepper

Salt and black pepper, to taste

4 Portobello mushrooms, cleaned and stemmed

2 tablespoons of onion slices

8 slices of bread

1 teaspoon of roasted garlic, mashed

5 teaspoons of mayonnaise

4 ounces of mozzarella cheese, sliced thinly

1 medium tomato, sliced

Fresh basil leaves, as required

Directions:

Preheat grill for medium-high heat. Grease the grate of grill. Grill red bell pepper for 10 to 12 minutes or till skin is charred from all sides. Let it cool.

Remove the skin and slice thinly. Keep aside.

In a small bowl, mix olive oil, salt and black pepper. Brush the mushrooms with seasoned oil. Grill mushrooms for about 3 minutes. Brush the mushrooms again with seasoned oil. Now grill mushrooms for 3 minutes more or till they become soft and juicy. Keep warm mushrooms in a plate.

Grill onion slices for 2 minutes per side. Toast the slices in grill for about 1 minute.

In a bowl, mix garlic and mayonnaise. In a medium bowl, mix bell peppers, mushrooms, onion, tomatoes and basil leaves.

Spread garlic mayonnaise on each slice. Place cheese slices. Spread mushroom mixture on slice. Cover with another slice, mayonnaise side down.

Serving Suggestions:

Serve as a side with salad or French fries.

Black Bean & Corn Wraps

These tasty and healthy wraps are yielded quickly and effortlessly.

Ingredients:

2 tablespoons of olive oil

2 cloves of garlic, minced

½ cup of canned black beans, rinsed and drained

¼ cup of frozen corns

Salt and black pepper, to taste

2 eggs

¼ teaspoon of red pepper flakes, crushed

½ teaspoon of cumin powder

¼ cup of mozzarella cheese, grated

2 large tortillas

2 tablespoons f sour cream

¼ cup of chopped lettuce leaves

6 cherry tomatoes, halved

Directions:

In a frying pan, heat oil on medium heat. Add garlic, beans and corns. Cook for 1 to 2 minutes. Season with some salt and black pepper. Transfer bean mixture to a plate.

Reduce heat to low. In a bowl, add eggs, pepper flakes, cumin and a pinch of salt. Whisk well. Spread egg mixture in the same frying pan evenly.

Sprinkle cheese and cook till cheese is melted and eggs are done completely. Cut eggs into strips.

Place tortillas in plate. Spread sour cream evenly. Place half of eggs and bean mixture on each tortilla. Add lettuce and tomatoes. Roll the tortillas. Place each tortilla in pan and toast for 30 seconds each side.

Serving Suggestions:

You can have a superb meal if these wraps are served alongside roasted carrots and potatoes.

Swiss Chard Wraps

These Swiss chard wraps sound like the perfect and fast vegetable-filled lunch.

Ingredients:

12 medium Swiss chard leaves, washed and stems removed

4 roma tomatoes, sliced

8 ounces of mozzarella cheese, sliced

1 red onion, diced

20 fresh basil leaves, chopped

Salt, to taste

Oil for brushing

Directions:

Steam chard halves till just wilted.

Place one of wilted chard halve on a cutting board. Place another half on first one cross wise. In center, place tomato slice, then cheese slice and top with onion and basil leaves. Sprinkle salt.

Wrap chard leaves in a bundle shape.

Preheat grill. Brush the grate of grill. Brush the outside of wraps.

Grill for 2 to 3 minutes per side.

Serving Suggestions:

Serve these wraps as a side dish with cooked rice.

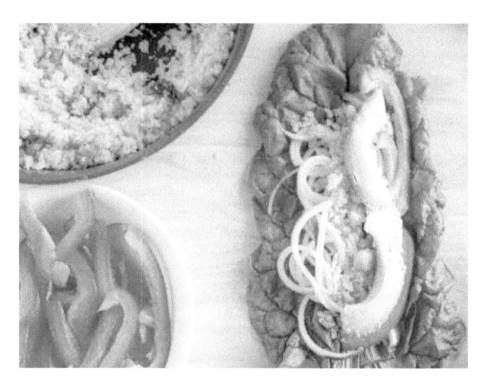

Tofu & White Beans Wraps

These yummy wraps have incredibly rich and flavorful filling.

Ingredients:

1 tablespoons of olive oil

4 tablespoons of fresh lime juice, divided

1 clove of garlic, minced

½ cup of red onion, chopped

¼ cup of fresh cilantro, chopped

8 ounces of firm tofu, drained, pat dried and crumbled

1 (15-ounce) can of white beans, rinsed, drained and mashed

Salt and black pepper, to taste

4 medium tortillas

2 cups of lettuce, sliced thinly

1 cup of prepared salsa

Directions:

Preheat oven to 350 degrees F.

In a bowl, add oil and 3 tablespoons of lime juice and whisk. Add garlic, onion, cilantro, tofu and beans. Season with salt and pepper. Toss to combine well. Keep aside for 20 minutes.

Fold tortillas in foil paper. Place in pre-heated oven for10 minutes.

In another bowl, toss lettuce and remaining lime juice.

Place tortilla in a plate. Spread layer of lettuce in center. Place tofu mixture on lettuce. Pour salsa on top and roll the tortillas.

Serving Suggestions:

Serve these wraps with tortilla chips.

Hummus Wraps

In these wraps, hummus and veggie salad make a nutritious and delicious meal-in-a-pocket.

Ingredients:

½ cup of mozzarella cheese, grated

1 medium tomato, chopped

1 small carrot, grated

¼ green bell pepper, diced finely

1 scallion, sliced thinly

1 cup of lettuce, shredded

Salt and black pepper, to taste

4 medium tortillas

4 tablespoons of hummus

Directions:

In a bowl, add all ingredients except tortillas and hummus and mix till well combined.

Spread hummus on each tortilla. Place vegetable mixture on hummus.

Roll up tortillas and serve.

Serving Suggestions:

Serve up these wraps with a side of potato salad.

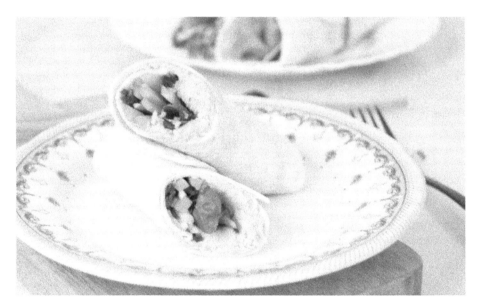

Peanut Butter & Banana Wraps

Sounds yummy...... Surely a great healthy breakfast for your kids!

Ingredients:

4 whole-wheat tortillas

½ cup of peanut butter

2 small bananas, sliced and dipped in orange juice

¼ cup of honey

¼ cup of semisweet chocolate chips

Directions:

Place tortilla in a plate.

Spread peanut butter on each tortilla evenly. Place banana slices. Pour 1 tablespoon of honey on banana slices. Sprinkle chocolate chips on top.

Roll up the tortillas.

Serving Suggestions:

Serve these yummy wraps with banana smoothie to your little ones in breakfast or snack time.

Garden Veggie Pita

This pita is a light but full of vegetable nutrient meal.

Ingredients:

½ cup of broccoli florets, chopped

½ cup of cauliflower florets, chopped

¼ cup of mushrooms, sliced

¼ cup of carrots, shredded

¼ cup of green bell pepper, chopped

¼ cup of red bell pepper, chopped

1 tablespoon of red onion, sliced finely

2 tablespoons of mayonnaise

1 teaspoon of Worcestershire sauce

1 teaspoon of lemon juice

¼ teaspoon of dried basil

Salt and black pepper, to taste

2 (6-inch) whole-wheat pita breads, halved

Directions:

In a bowl, add all vegetables and toss well.

In another bowl, add mayonnaise, Worcestershire sauce, lemon juice, basil, salt and black pepper and mix well.

Mix vegetables and mayonnaise mixture and toss to coat well.

Place the vegetable mixture in each half of pita bread.

Serving Suggestions:

Serve with pita chips.

Falafel Pitas

These pitas are easy to prepare and having nice crunchy exterior and zesty flavor!!

Ingredients:

For Patties:

1 (15-ounce) can of chickpeas, rinsed and drained

¼ cup of plain dry breadcrumbs

¼ cup of red onion, minced

2 egg whites

1 slice of whole-wheat bread, torn into small pieces

Salt and black pepper, to taste

½ teaspoon of paprika

1 teaspoon of cumin powder

1 tablespoon of Dijon mustard

1½ tablespoons of canola oil

For Pitas:

2 (6-inch) whole-wheat pitas, halved

4 lettuce leaves

8 tomato slices

½ cup of cucumber-yogurt dressing

Directions:

Preheat oven to 350 degrees F.

In a food processor, add all patties ingredients except oil and blend till well mixed.

In a large frying pan, heat oil on medium-high heat. Make patties from chickpeas mixture. Place patties in pan and cook for 4 minutes from each side or till they become golden brown.

Open the pita bread to make pockets. Toast for 10 minutes or till crispy and light brown.

Line each pita pocket with tomato slices and lettuce leaves. Stuff the pitas with patties.

Drizzle with dressing generously over patties.

Serving Suggestions:

Serve falafel pitas with fresh crunchy salad.

Hummus & Chickpeas Pitas

These pitas are healthy option that you can throw together for a tasty lunch.

Ingredients:

2 tablespoons of olive oil,

2 (15-ounce) cans of chickpeas, rinsed and drained

Salt and black pepper, to taste

¼ cup of fresh parsley, chopped

4 (6-inch) whole-wheat pitas, halved and warmed

1 (8-ounce) jar of hummus

1 red onion, sliced thinly

1 teaspoon of Tabasco sauce

Directions:

In a skillet, heat oil on medium-high heat. Add chickpeas. Cook, stirring for about 5 minutes or until they become light brown. Remove from stove.

Stir in salt, black pepper and parsley and mix well.

Spread hummus in pita halves. Place chickpeas mixture.

Top with onion slices and Tabasco sauce.

Serving Suggestions:

Serve these pitas with yogurt dip and lemon wedges.

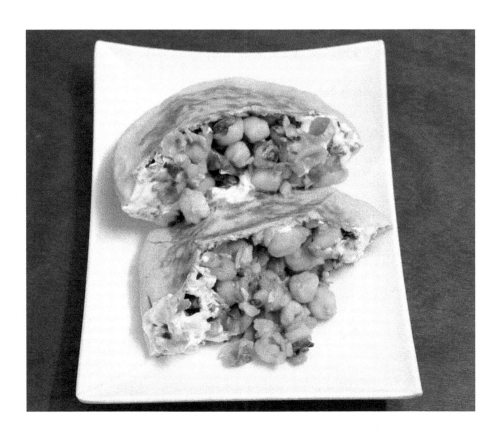

Avocado & Tomato Pitas

These pitas are easy, tasty and nutrient packed...

Ingredients:

½ cup of mayonnaise

¼ cup of Parmesan cheese, grated

½ teaspoon of sugar

1 teaspoon of lemon juice

Salt and black pepper, to taste

1 large tomato, sliced

1 avocado, sliced

2 (6-inch) whole-wheat pitas, halved and toasted

Directions:

In a bowl, add mayonnaise, cheese, sugar, lemon juice, salt and black pepper and mix well.

Spread mayonnaise dressing on each half of pitas.

Then place tomato and avocado slices and serve.

Serving Suggestions:

These pitas will be more flavorful if served with fresh fruit salad.

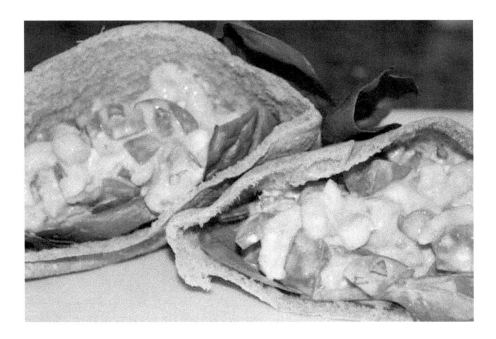

Mediterranean Vegetable Pitas

Here is a delicious and healthy pita sandwich, hearty enough for light dinner too.

Ingredients:

2 tablespoons of extra-virgin olive oil

¼ teaspoons of garlic powder

Cayenne pepper powder, to taste

½ teaspoon of fresh oregano, chopped

1 teaspoon of lemon peel, grated

¼ cup of feta cheese, crumbled

¼ cup of ripe olives, pitted and chopped

½ cup of tomato, chopped finely

¼ cup of red onion, chopped finely

½ cup of cucumber, chopped finely

¾ cup of lettuce leaves, sliced thinly

4 (6-inch) whole-grain pitas, halved

Directions:

In a bowl, add oil, garlic powder, cayenne pepper powder, oregano and lemon peel. Mix till well combined.

Stir in remaining ingredients except pita halves and mix gently.

Place vegetable mixture in pita halves and serve.

Serving Suggestions:

Complete and yummy meal if served with tomato soup.

Roasted Veggie Pinwheels

These colorful and tasty pinwheels are perfect as an appetizer or snack......

Ingredients:

2 large green bell peppers

2 large red bell peppers

2 large yellow bell peppers

1 (15-ounce) can of chickpeas, rinsed and drained

6 tablespoons of water

¼ cup of fresh lemon juice

½ cup of tahini sauce

1 clove of garlic

Salt, to taste

1½ cucumber, peeled, seeded and sliced thinly

3 large carrots, peeled And sliced thinly

6 (10-inch) whole wheat tortillas

Directions:

Preheat oven to 325 degrees F.

Place bell peppers on greased cookie sheet. Roast bell peppers for 10 to 15 minutes. Let them cool.

Peel and remove seeds. Cut into slices.

In a food processor, add chickpeas, water, lemon juice, tahini sauce, garlic and salt and blend till smooth.

Transfer chickpeas mixture to a bowl.

Place tortillas in plates. Spread chickpeas mixture on tortillas evenly. Place cucumber and carrots on mixture. Roll up the tortillas.

Wrap in plastic bags and refrigerate for at least 3 hours.

While serving, remove plastic bags and trim the ends. Then cut into 1-inch slices and serve.

Serving Suggestions:

These pinwheels work great as a soup partner.

Cream Cheese & Olives Pinwheels

Olives and scallions give an interesting texture and flavor to pinwheels.

Ingredients:

1 (8-ounce) package of cream cheese

2 teaspoons of cayenne pepper sauce

1 cup of black olives, pitted and chopped

4 scallions, chopped

6 (10-inch) flour tortillas

Directions:

In a bowl, add all ingredients except tortillas and mix till well combined.

Spread a thin and even layer on each tortilla.

Roll up each tortilla in plastic wraps and refrigerate for at least 1 hour.

Just before serving, remove plastic wraps and cut the ends. Then cut into 1-inch slices.

Serving Suggestions:

Have a full meal lunch with the combination of these pinwheels and salad.

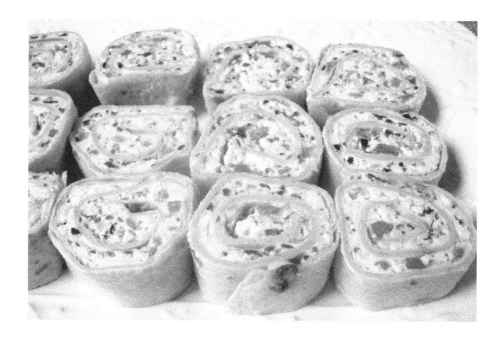

Nacho Cheese Pinwheels

These pinwheels are easy and quick addition to an appetizer plate.

Ingredients:

4 (8-inch) flour tortillas

½ cup of nacho cheese dip

½ cup of bean dip

2 tablespoons of scallions, chopped

2 tablespoons of cilantro, chopped

Directions:

Place tortillas on plates.

Spread cheese and bean dip evenly on each tortilla. Top with chopped scallion and cilantro.

Roll up tortillas in plastic bags. Refrigerate to chill for about 1 hour.

While serving remove plastic bags and trim the ends. Cut into 1-inch slices.

Serving Suggestions:

Serve with salsa and sour cream.

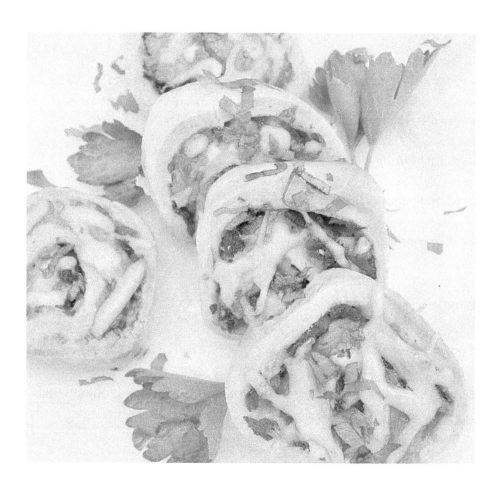

Cranberry & Feta Cheese Pinwheels

These are versatile and best flavored snacks for special occasions.

Ingredients:

1 cup of feta cheese, crumbled

1 (8-ounce) package of cream cheese, whipped

¼ cup of scallions, chopped finely

1 (6-ounce) package of dried cranberries

4 (8-inch) wheat tortillas

Directions:

In a bowl, add feta cheese, cream cheese and scallions and mix till well combined. Fold in cranberries. Spread cranberry mixture evenly on each tortilla.

Roll up in plastic wraps and refrigerate for about 1 hour.

Just before serving remove plastic wraps and trim the ends. Then cut into 1-inch slices.

Serving Suggestions:

For more sweetness and colors you can spread an extra layer of pepper jelly on tortilla.

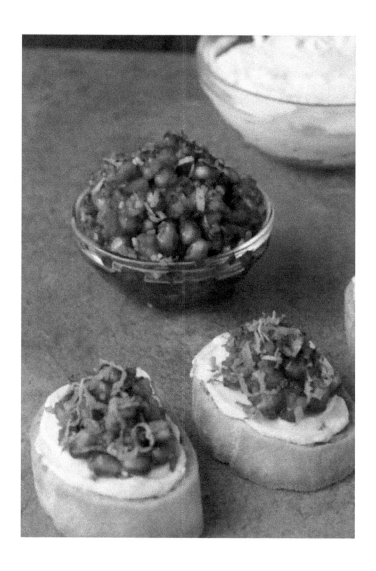

Spinach & Swiss Cheese Pinwheels

Here is a great tasting and good looking appetizer!!

Ingredients:

1 tablespoon of sour cream

1 (8-ounce) package of cream cheese, whipped

1 teaspoon of fennel seeds, crushed

2 tablespoons of onion, minced

2 medium tomatoes, sliced thinly

4 cups of spinach, torn

¼ cup of olives, pitted and sliced thinly

10 slices of Swiss cheese

6 (8-inch) wheat tortillas

Directions:

In a bowl, add sour cream, cream cheese, fennel seeds and onions and mix till combined.

In another bowl mix remaining ingredients except tortillas.

Spread cream cheese mixture on tortillas. Top with Swiss cheese mixture. Roll up the tortillas and wrap in plastic bags.

Refrigerate at least for 4 hours.

Just before serving, remove the plastic bags and cut the ends. Cut into 1-inch slices.

Serving Suggestions:

These pinwheels are great if served with a creamy dressing.

White Beans Burgers

A mild yet flavorful burger!!

Ingredients:

2 cups of white beans, cooked

1 large red onion, minced

1 clove of garlic, minced

1 (4.5-ounce) can of green chilies, chopped

1 egg

Salt and black pepper, to taste

1 teaspoon of cumin powder

1 cup of breadcrumbs

2 tablespoons of olive oil

Mozzarella cheese, sliced, as required

Lettuce leaves, as required

4 burger buns, toasted

Directions:

In a food processor, add beans and blend till mashed slightly. Transfer to a bowl. Now add onion, garlic, green chilies, egg, salt, black pepper, cumin and breadcrumbs. Mix till well combined. Make patties from mixture.

Refrigerate for 20 minutes.

In a frying pan, heat oil on medium heat. Place patties over pan and cook for 4 to 5 minutes per side or till golden brown.

Place patties in buns with cheese slices and lettuce leaves.

Serving Suggestions:

Serve this burger in a platter with a side of steamed vegetables.

Fava Bean Burgers

Fava beans burger is just what you need for a healthy meal.

Ingredients:

4 tablespoons of canola oil, divided

½ cup of onion, chopped finely

1 teaspoon of garlic, minced

¼ teaspoon of cayenne pepper

½ teaspoon of coriander powder

¾ teaspoon of cumin powder

1 ¾ cups of fresh fava beans, shelled and peeled

Salt and black pepper, to taste

2 tablespoons of tahini sauce

1 large egg

4 burger buns, toasted

Lettuce leaves, as required

1 large tomato, sliced

Directions:

In a large pan, heat 1 tablespoon of oil on medium heat. Sauté onion for 4 to 5 minutes.

Stir in garlic, cayenne pepper, coriander and cumin. Cook for 1 minute. Transfer into a bowl.

In a food processor, add fava beans and pulse till chopped coarsely. Add ½ cup of chopped fava into onion mixture.

In the same food processor, add salt, pepper, tahini sauce and egg and pulse again till well combined. Then mix in onion mixture.

Make patties from mixture. In a frying pan, heat remaining oil on medium heat.

Cook patties for 3 minutes each side or till golden and crisp. Place patties in burger buns. Top with lettuce leaves.

Serving Suggestions:

Enjoy this delicious burger with potato wedges and salad.

Greek Lentil Burgers

Fabulous recipe! Absolutely your kids will love it.

Ingredients:

For patties:

3¼ cups of green lentils, cooked according to package directions

Salt, to taste

4 large eggs

½ teaspoon of black pepper

1 clove of garlic

1 onion, chopped finely

1 tablespoon of fresh dill, chopped finely

2 tablespoons of fresh mint, chopped finely

1 cup of breadcrumbs, toasted slightly

2 tablespoons of olive oil

For burgers:

4 burger buns, toasted

Lettuce leaves

Onion slices

Tomato slices

Swiss cheese slices

Directions:

In a food processor, add lentils, salt and egg and blend till smooth. Transfer to a bowl.

Add remaining ingredients except oil and mix till well combined.

Make patties from mixture.

In a frying pan, heat oil on medium heat. Cook patties for 4 to 5 minutes per side or till crispy and brown.

Place patties in burger buns. Top with lettuce, tomato, onion and cheese slices.

Serving Suggestions:

Enjoy your burger with potato salad.

Tofu Burgers

A spectacular burger for anyone looking for something different...

Ingredients:

1 (12-ounces) package of firm tofu, drained and pat dried

5 tablespoons of canola oil

1 egg, beaten

1 small onion, chopped

1 tablespoon of garlic, minced

1 stalk of celery, minced

1 teaspoon of cumin powder

Salt and pepper, to taste

¼ cup of cheddar cheese, shredded

¼ cup of breadcrumbs

4 sesame seeds burger buns

Lettuce leaves

Tomato slices

Onion slices

Directions:

In a bowl, add tofu and mash with a fork.

In a pan, heat 1 tablespoon of oil on medium heat. Sauté onion, garlic and celery till golden brown. Transfer to tofu bowl.

Now add remaining ingredients and mix till ell combined.

Make patties from mixture. In a non-stick frying pan, heat remaining oil on medium-high heat. Cook patties for 5 to7 minutes per side or till golden.

Place patties in burger buns. Top with lettuce, tomato and onion slices.

Serving Suggestions:

Serve this spectacular and tasty burger with watermelon soda.

Mushroom & Barley Burgers

The combination of mushrooms and barley makes deliciously chewy ad nutty tasting burger.

Ingredients:

4 tablespoons of olive oil, divided

2 cups of onion, chopped finely

½ pound of cremini mushrooms, chopped finely

2 tablespoons of garlic, minced

2 tablespoons of balsamic vinegar

3 cups of barley, cooked

4 eggs, beaten

Salt and black pepper, to taste

½ cup of walnuts, roasted and chopped finely

1 cup of mozzarella cheese, grated

4 soft burger buns

Lettuce leaves

Directions:

In a skillet, heat 1 tablespoon of oil on medium-high heat. Sauté onion for about 5 minutes or till translucent.

Add garlic and mushrooms. Cook, stirring for 10 minutes or till liquid is absorbed. Remove from stove and stir in the vinegar.

In a bowl, add mushroom mixture, barley, eggs, salt, black pepper, walnuts and cheese. Mix till well combined.

Keep aside for 15 minutes. Make patties from the mixture.

In a non-stick frying pan, heat remaining oil on medium heat.

Cook patties for 4 to 5 minutes per side or till golden brown.

Place patties in buns and top with lettuce.

Serving Suggestions:

Enjoy these delicious burgers with vegan mayonnaise.

Onion & Tomato Pizza

A very easy to prepare recipe that even your kids would love to help you.

Ingredients:

1 pizza base

3 tablespoons of pizza sauce

2 packages of cheddar cheese, sliced

1 green bell pepper, chopped

2 medium tomatoes, chopped

2 green chilies, chopped finely

2 red onions, sliced in rings

1 package of mozzarella cheese, grated

1 teaspoon of oregano

1 teaspoon of salt

½ teaspoon of black pepper powder

Directions:

Preheat oven to 375 degrees F. Line a baking dish with wax paper.

Place the pizza base on baking dish. Spread pizza paste on base evenly.

Place cheese slices on it. Place bell pepper on cheese. Then place tomato and green chilies. Now place onion rings. Spread grated cheese on vegetables. Sprinkle oregano, salt and black pepper.

Place pizza in oven and bake for about 10 - 12 minutes.

Serving Suggestions:

Enjoy with a side salad.

Four Cheese Pizza

The rich combination of cheese adds a superb flavor that brings this pizza to life.

Ingredients:

1½ tablespoons of extra-virgin olive oil

¼ teaspoon of salt

½ tablespoon of garlic, minced

4 roman tomatoes, sliced

1 Boboli pre-cooked pizza crust

2 ounces of Fontina cheese, shredded

8 ounces of mozzarella cheese, shredded

5 fresh basil leaves

¼ cup of feta cheese, crumbled

¼ cup of Parmesan cheese, grated

Directions:

Preheat oven to 400 degrees F. Line a baking dish with wax paper.

In a bowl, add oil, salt, garlic and tomatoes and toss to coat well. Keep aside for 10 minutes.

Place pizza crust on baking dish. Grease pizza crust with a little tomato marinade.

Place Fontina and mozzarella cheese evenly. Spread tomato mixture on cheese. Now place basil leaves. Top with feta and Parmesan cheese.

Bake for 10 minutes or till cheese become golden brown and bubbly.

Serving Suggestions:

Enjoy cheesy pizza with faro salad.

Garden Vegetables Pizza

Surely it can be a family favorite pizza.

Ingredients:

2 tablespoons of extra-virgin olive oil

1 large squash, diced

1 large zucchini, diced

1 small eggplant, diced

1 onion, diced

2 cloves of garlic, minced

2 medium tomatoes, diced

½ teaspoon of salt

¼ teaspoon of black pepper powder

2 sprigs of fresh thyme, chopped

1 sprig of fresh oregano, chopped

6 fresh basil leaves, chopped

1 pre-cooked pizza crust

1½ cups of mozzarella cheese, shredded

1 cup of Parmesan cheese, grated

Directions:

Preheat oven to 400 degrees F.

Line a baking dish with wax paper.

In a skillet, heat oil on medium heat. Add squash, zucchini and eggplant. Cook, stirring for about 8 to 10 minutes or till tender.

Add onion, garlic, tomato, salt and black pepper. Cook for 3 minutes more. Add fresh herbs and remove from stove immediately.

Place pizza crust in baking dish. Sprinkle 1 cup of mozzarella cheese on pizza crust.

Spread vegetable mixture on cheese. Sprinkle remaining mozzarella and Parmesan cheese on top. Bake for 8 to 10 minutes.

Serving Suggestions:

Serve with sour cream.

Spinach & Mozzarella Cheese Pizza

Yummy!! Surely your family would love this healthier and tasty pizza.

Ingredients:

1 large tomato, sliced

1 tablespoon of garlic, chopped finely

1 pre-cooked pizza crust

3 cups of fresh spinach, chopped

Italian seasoning, as required

1 cup of mozzarella cheese, grated

Directions:

Preheat oven to 400 degrees F.

Line a baking sheet with wax paper. Mix well tomatoes and garlic.

Place pizza crust in baking dish. Spread tomato slices on crust. Now place spinach on tomatoes. Sprinkle Italian seasoning on vegetables. Top with grated cheese.

Bake for 8 to 10 minutes.

Serving Suggestions:

Have a complete meal of yummy pizza sided with fresh salad.

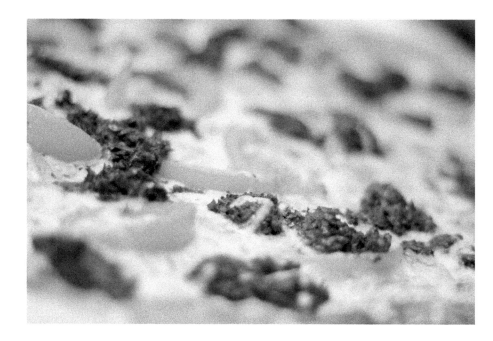

Black Bean & Corn Pizza

It will be a big hit for friends get together.

Ingredients:

1 cup of fresh corn kernels

1 cup of black beans, cooked

1 plum tomato, chopped

1 pre-cooked pizza crust

1/3 cup of barbecue sauce

1 cup of mozzarella cheese, shredded

Directions:

Preheat oven to 450 degrees F.

Line a baking sheet with wax paper. Place crust on baking sheet. Spread barbecue sauce on crust evenly.

Place beans mixture on sauce. Top with cheese.

Bake for 7 minutes or till crust is browned and cheese is melted.

Serving Suggestions:

Have more fun by eating your pizza with fresh veggie salad.

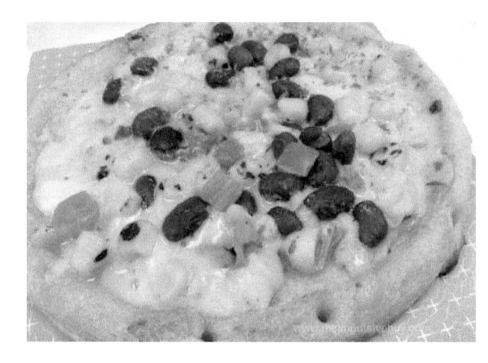

Carrot & Celery Soup

Ingredients:

2 tablespoons of olive oil plus a little more for drizzling

4 carrots, peeled and sliced

4 celery stalks, washed and sliced thinly

1 onion, chopped

5 cloves of garlic, minced finely

8 cups of vegetable broth

1 large celery root, peeled and cubed (just before adding)

1½ teaspoons of dill seed

Salt and black pepper, to taste

Directions:

In a large pan, heat oil on medium-high heat.

Add carrots, celery and onion. Sprinkle with salt and sauté for about 5 minutes.

Now add garlic and sauté for 1 minute.

Add broth and bring to a boil. Now add celery root and dill seeds. Cook for 20 to 30 minutes, or until vegetables are tender.

Season with salt and black pepper.

Puree soup in a blender till smooth. While serving, drizzle a little olive oil over soup.

Serving Suggestions:

Serve this soup with toasted and chopped peanuts to have even more great flavor.

Lightning Source UK Ltd.
Milton Keynes UK
UKHW020631190821
389117UK00013B/1036